The Updated IC Diet Cookbook

The Essential Guide with Healthy and Delicous
Breakfast, Lunch, Dinner and Dessert Recipes to
Treat Interstitial Cystitis Symptoms, Bladder
Pain And Relief Pelvic

D0833541

Table of Contents

DISCLAIMER

Please note that the information and recipes in this book are written for the express purpose of sharing educational information only. The information herein is stated to be reliable and consistence, but the author neither implies nor intends any guarantee of accuracy for specific cases or individuals.

It is recommended that you consult a licensed professional before beginning any practise relating to your diet or lifestyle. The contents of this book are not replacement for professional advice.

The author, publisher and distributors disclaim any liability, loss or damage and risk taken by individuals who directly or indirectly act on the information contained in this book.

Introduction

Interstitial cystitis (IC) is a chronic bladder condition which often presents with pelvic pain, urinary urgency and urinary frequency. Although this sounds very similar to a bacterial bladder infection, this chronic condition is not caused by an infection. The diagnosis is established by exclusion of other conditions such as infection, bladder stones, kidney disease, sexually transmitted diseases, endometriosis, and other disorders. Sometimes, a camera into the urinary bladder called cystoscopy is performed to look for red patches or other abnormalities that can be seen with the camera.

IC is often associated with other concomitant diseases. In our practice we see IC can coexist with endometriosis, allergies, irritable bowel syndrome, fibromyalgia, inflammatory bowel disease (Crohn's disease and ulcerative colitis), and Sjögren's syndrome. Often, the treatment for the underlying conditions helps the IC improve as well. We usually start with dietary changes (such as removing acidic food, citrus fruits and coffee from the diet). If that is not helpful, the specialist can recommend medications, supplements, psychosocial support, pelvic floor therapy, and biofeedback.

Symptoms of Interstitial Cystitis

- The frequent and urgent need to urinate

- Pain or pressure in the bladder area, often relieved for a short time after urinating
- Pain in the genitals or anus
- Painful sexual intercourse
- Symptoms in women may get worse during their period. Symptoms may go away for a period of time (remission), but they often come back again.

Causes of interstitial cystitis

Although the symptoms of interstitial cystitis are similar to those of a chronic urinary tract infection, bacteria are rarely found in patient urine samples.

While the true cause of interstitial cystitis is unknown, there are several theories as to what causes the condition. Some possible causes include:

- Defects in the epithelium (lining) of the urinary bladder causing irritation
- Bladder trauma or overdistention
- Pelvic floor muscle dysfunction
- Autoimmune disorders
- Primary neurogenic inflammation
- Spinal cord trauma
- Genetics or heredity
- Allergy.

Treatment For Interstitial Cystitis

Specific treatment for IC will be determined by your doctor based on:

- Your age, overall health, and medical history
- Extent of the disease
- The presence of an ulcer in the bladder
- Your tolerance for specific medications, procedures, or therapies
- Expectations for the course of the disease
- Your opinion or preference

Often times more than one treatment is necessary to optimally treat IC/BPS. In general your doctor will usually recommend the simplest treatments first. Treatments are primarily focused on relieving symptoms, and may include:

- **Lifestyle and Dietary Changes:** There are many self-care practices and behavioral modifications that can be used to improve symptoms. Stress management has been shown to help some patients with IC/BPS. For some women, symptoms can be triggered by certain activities of food/drinks. If these can be identified, reducing or eliminating them can be very helpful. Some patients respond well to an IC diet where many acid foods are eliminated.

- **Physical Therapy:** Appropriate manual physical therapy techniques that are designed to reduce pelvic pain may be performed by trained clinicians. Pelvic floor strengthening exercises should be avoided.

- **Medications:** There are a number of oral medications that may be helpful for some patients. These may be tried alone or in combination.

- **Bladder instillations:** The bladder is filled with one of several solutions that are held for varying periods of time.

- **Cystoscopy with hydrodistension:** In some women, the bladder can be filled under anesthesia for a period of time under low pressure. This has been found be relieve symptoms is some patients who have not responded to behavioral therapy, physical therapy or medication.

- **Cystoscopy with fulguration of a Hunner's lesion:** If a Hunner's lesion or ulcer is identified with cystoscopy fulguration with laser or electrocautery may be recommended. This has a high likelihood of resolving pain.

- **Botulinum Toxin:** In rare circumstances you doctor may recommend that you consider Botox injections into the bladder when other conventional treatments have not worked.

- **Sacral Neuromodulation:** Sacral neuromodulation or Interstim where the nerves to the bladder are stimulated with an electric current supplied by an implanted device or "pacemaker" may be considered in cases when other conventional treatments have not worked.

- **Reconstructive Surgery:** This may be considered as a last resort for some women with severe IC/BPS that has not responded to other treatments.

Interstitial Cystitis and Diet

Interstitial Cystitis (IC) is not well understood but the link between food and the occurrence of pain episodes is very clear. The list of foods that can irritate the bladder and thus cause pelvic pain in patients with IC is long. The important point is that not every food on the list will be an issue for every patient. As in the case of most situations, every person is unique and will respond differently to different foods.

Though, Most patients with Interstitial Cystitis will notice a significant decrease in pain severity and episodes after following these diet rules.

Foods That Can Hurt The Bladder

CAFFEINE

Caffeine acts as a diuretic, stimulating more frequent urination and also causes urine to become more concentrated with urea and ammonia. All caffeinated products (coffees, teas, green teas, energy drinks, etc.) should be stopped immediately.

ACIDIC FOODS

Foods high in acid (i.e. citrus fruits and juices, cranberry, vinegar) create irritation in much the same way that acid poured on a wound on your hand would feel. It hurts! Cranberries, for example, contain quinic, malic and citric acid which may help us understand why cranberry juice is irritating for most of us.

ALCOHOL

In an ICN Survey, beer, wine and spirits bothered roughly 95% patients though there is some wiggle room with lower acid varieties.

POTASSIUM

11

Some, but not all, patients may struggle with high potassium foods though research studies have found that bananas and yams, both high in potassium, are usually bladder soothing. Try small amounts of high potassium foods to see if you tolerate them well.

HISTAMINE

Researchers have found that the bladders of IC patients have high numbers of activated mast cells. These mast cells have released histamine which then provokes an allergic reaction in the bladder, triggering frequency, urgency and/or pain. Not surprisingly, foods high in histamine, such as chocolate and red wine, are well known to trigger bladder discomfort.

ARTIFICIAL SWEETENERS

Both research studies and patient stories have confirmed that most artificial sweeteners (aspartame, saccharin, sucralose, etc.) appear to be bladder irritating, particularly aspartame (i.e. NutraSweet®). Most diet products, such as sugar free iced tea or soda, should be avoided.

MSG, NITRITES & NITRATES

MSG is a mast cell degranulator and for patients sensitive or allergic to it, can cause rash, hives, asthma and sudden diarrhea known as"Chinese restaurant syndrome." IC patients have long reported that foods containing high levels of MSG and/or nitrates trigger bladder symptoms and discomfort, thus we suggest avoiding these foods whenever possible.

VITAMINS & SUPPLEMENTS

Both patients and research report that multivitamins can trigger bladder symptoms due, most likely, to high levels of Vitamin C (ascorbic acid) and Vitamin B6. Unless you have a medical condition that requires using a multivitamin, we suggest that you avoid vitamin supplements and waters in favor of eating fresh foods and vegetables. If you need a multivitamin, we suggest trying MultiRight, a low acid multivitamin and mineral complex that the IC Network helped to develop. It works well for most patients.

CHOCOLATE

Chocolate contains several ingredients that have the potential to exacerbate IC symptoms: theobromine, caffeine, phenylethylamine, tannins and oxalates. Well known for triggering migraine headaches, IC patients often report flares from eating chocolates, particularly cheaper milk chocolate products

GLUTEN

In The Better Bladder Book, author Wendy Cohen was the first to suggest that gluten could be irritating some patients. It's worth experimenting with gluten free products to determine if gluten could be a source of irritation.

Healthy and Delicious IC Diet Recipes

Slow Cooker Potato Soup

Ingredients

- 1 (30 oz.) bag frozen hash-brown potatoes (I use the squared, southern style)
- 2 (14 oz.) cans chicken broth (regular or low-sodium)
- 1 (10.75 oz.) can cream of potato soup
- 1/4 tsp. ground black pepper
- 1/4 tsp. onion powder, if desired

- 1 (8 oz.) block cream cheese (very softened)
- Chopped scallions (green onion), if desired

Instructions

1. In a slow cooker, combine potatoes, broth, soup and pepper. (Honestly, I don't usually measure the pepper. I just do a few turns on the pepper grinder and call it good.) Add a dash of onion powder, if desired.

2. Cover, and cook on low for 4 hours.

3. Stir in cream cheese, cook another 45 minutes to 1 hour, stirring occasionally, until combined.

4. Top each bowl with shredded cheese and bacon bits (or crispy bacon). Add

some chopped scallions, if desired. Enjoy!

Tomatoless Lasagne

Servings: 8

Ingredients

- 1 pkg. frozen chopped spinach (10 oz.)
- 3/4 cup grated carrots
- 1-1/4 cups grated zucchini squash
- 1/4 cup feta cheese, crumbled
- 1-1/4 cup grated low-fat mozzarella
- 4 cups (32 oz carton) cottage cheese, divided
- 1 egg
- 2 tsp. dried chives (optional if they bother you)
- 1 pkg. lasagne noodles (approx 16 oz.)

- 3-1/2 cups Campbell's Healthy Request or Nature Valley chicken broth
- 1/2 cup flour
- 1/2 tsp. nutmeg
- 1 Tbsp. olive oil
- extra grated mozzarella

Instructions

1. In a large bowl, stir together the spinach, carrots, zucchini, feta cheese, mozzarella, and 3 cups of the cottage cheese. Stir in the egg and dried chives. Set aside. Cook the pasta noodles according to the package directions.

2. While the noodles cook, stir together in a large saucepan the broth, flour, nutmeg and remaining cottage cheese. Cook while stirring until mixture

comes to a boil. Remove from heat.
Drain noodles.

3. Brush or wipe bottom of a 13 x 9 inch
baking dish with olive oil. Spread with
a little sauce.

4. Layer the dish beginning with pasta
noodles, then vegetable mixture, then
sauce. Repeat layers, then top with
final layer of noodles. Spread
remainder of sauce on top. Top with a
little extra grated mozzarella. Cover
with foil and bake at 350 degrees F. for
45 minutes or until bubbly hot.
Remove, uncover, and let stand 8-10
minutes before serving.

Shepherd's Pie

Ingredients

- 1 lb lean (at least 80%) ground beef
- 1 medium onion, chopped (1 cup) (if tolerated)
- 2 medium carrots, peeled, chopped (1 cup)
- 2 tablespoons all-purpose flour
- 1 1/2 teaspoons finely chopped fresh thyme leaves
- 1/2 teaspoon salt
- 1/4 teaspoon pepper (if tolerated)
- 1 cup chicken broth
- 1/2 cup frozen peas
- 1/2 cup frozen corn
- 1 (4.7 oz.) pouch creamy butter mashed potatoes

Instructions

1. Heat oven to 400°F. Spray 8-inch square (2-quart) glass baking dish with cooking spray.

2. In 12-inch nonstick skillet, cook beef over medium-high heat 4 minutes, stirring frequently. Add onion and carrots; cook 4 to 6 minutes, stirring occasionally, until beef is browned and onion and carrots are softened. Add flour, thyme, salt and pepper; cook 1 minute, stirring frequently.

3. Gradually stir in broth; heat to boiling over medium-high heat. Cook until thickened, stirring frequently. Remove from heat; stir in frozen peas and corn; transfer mixture to baking dish.

4. Make mashed potatoes as directed on pouch. Spread potatoes evenly over mixture in baking dish. Bake 20 to 25

minutes or until heated through (165°F in center) and top is lightly browned. Let stand 10 minutes before serving.

5. To freeze: Cook beef filling as directed in recipe, but do not add frozen peas and corn. Cover and refrigerate 30 to 40 minutes. Transfer to 1-quart freezer container; freeze up to 2 months. To bake: Heat oven to 400°F. Spray microwavable 8-inch square (2-quart) glass baking dish with cooking spray. Place frozen beef filling container in large bowl filled with hot water about 5 minutes or until filling can be slid out of container into 8-inch square dish. Cover with plastic wrap; microwave on High 5 minutes; stir well. Cover and microwave 3 minutes longer; stir well. Continue heating

another 3 to 4 minutes (checking and stirring every minute) until heated through. Stir in frozen peas and corn. Continue as directed in recipe.

Chicken Casserole

Servings: 4

Ingredients

- 2 tablespoons butter or margarine
- 5 tablespoons all-purpose flour
- 1-1/4 cups chicken broth (low-sodium, MSG-free), divided
- 1 cup milk
- 1/2 teaspoon salt (omit if using broth that's not low-sodium)
- 1/8 teaspoon garlic powder
- 1 dash white pepper (optional)

- 1/3 medium red onion, chopped & pre-fried as above (or 1 tsp. onion powder)
- 1-1/2 cups half-inch size, soft bread cubes (or cornbread crumbs or cooked pasta noodles)
- 1/2 cup finely chopped celery
- 2 tablespoons frozen peas or frozen carrots (optional)
- 3 cups cooked chicken, chopped
- 1 tablespoon chopped fresh chives
- 1 tablespoon Panko bread crumbs (optional)
- Non-stick cooking spray

Instructions

1. In a medium saucepan melt the butter. Remove from the heat and stir in the flour until it is all absorbed. Return the

pan to low heat and gradually stir in 1 cup of the chicken broth and all the milk until the sauce is thickened (don't boil). Stir in the salt, garlic powder, pepper and onion (or onion powder). Remove from the heat.

2. Preheat oven to 350 degrees F. Combine bread cubes, cornbread crumbs, or noodles with the chopped celery in a bowl. Pour the remaining 1/4-cup of chicken broth over the mixture and gently toss. Spray a 10-inch square or 12×8-inch casserole dish with non-stick cooking spray. Place half the chicken pieces in the bottom of the dish. Cover with half the celery mixture. Sprinkle on the frozen peas or carrots. Top with the remaining chicken, then the remaining celery

mixture. Pour the sauce over all and sprinkle the top with chopped chives and Panko crumbs (if desired).

3. Cover with foil or a heat-proof lid and bake at 350 degrees F. until hot and bubbly, about 30 to 35 minutes.

Baked Quesadillas

Ingredients

- Flour or wheat tortilla shells (soft taco or burrito size, depending on how big you want your quesadillas to be), 2 per quesadilla
- Spray margarine (can also use melted margarine or butter or, in a pinch, non-stick cooking spray)
- Shredded Mexican blend cheese
- Shredded Italian blend cheese

- Quesadilla fillings, such as bacon, chicken, ground beef, steak, onions, peppers, tomatoes, etc.

Instructions

1. Preheat the oven to 400-degrees.
2. Prepare baking sheets with non-stick cooking spray or line them with parchment paper or silicone baking mats.
3. Get out one tortilla shells per quesadilla. Cover on side of it with the margarine or butter. (For spray margarine, I use 8 to 10 squirts and smear it around with my clean hands.)
4. Please the shells buttered side down onto your prepared baking sheet(s).
5. Put your filling ingredients onto the top of the shells. Top them with

cheese. I use 3/4 Mexican blend or colby jack cheese and 1/4 Italian blend or mozzarella cheese. The amount of cheese varies based on the size of your shell and your family's preferences.

6. Then add whatever ingredients your family prefers. I love chicken bacon ranch using precooked, refrigerated chicken, precooked bacon cooked until crispy in the microwave, shredded cheese, ranch dressing, tomato, onion and roughly chopped spinach.

7. Place another tortilla on top. Lightly cover it with margarine or butter, just as you did the bottom shells.

8. Place into your preheated oven for 6 minutes.

9. Pull out the quesadillas and carefully flip them over.

10. Bake for 6 more minutes or until the edges are a nice golden brown.

11. Use a pizza cutter or sharp knife to slice and serve hot. We usually serve ours with sour cream because we love it!

Potatis (Swedish-style baked potatoes)

Servings: 2

Ingredients

- 2 medium-sized baking potatoes
- 3 Tbsp. melted butter or stick margarine
- Salt
- 1 Tbsp. grated Parmesan cheese or
- 2 Tbsp. grated Mozzarella cheese (see note)

- 2 Tbsp. dry bread crumbs from wheat bread
- extra butter or margarine

Instructions

1. Preheat the oven to 425 degrees F. Peel the potatoes. Carefully make slices across the potatoes, cutting only about three-quarters of the way through the potatoes. Leave the bottom half inch or so of the potato uncut. Make many thin cuts, one about every 1/8 inch. Place the potatoes uncut side down in a buttered baking dish. Pour the melted butter over the potatoes, allowing it to run between the slices. Sprinkle with salt.

2. Bake uncovered for 20 minutes at 425 degrees F. With a brush, brush the

potatoes with the butter in the pan. Bake another 20 minutes and brush the potatoes again with butter. Sprinkle potatoes with crumbs and cheese. Bake another 5 minutes. Remove and allow to cool 5 minutes before serving.

Swedish Meatballs

Servings: 3

Ingredients

Meatballs:

- 1 egg
- 3/4 tsp. ground nutmeg
- 3/4 tsp. ground allspice
- 1/4 tsp. salt
- 1 lb. lean ground beef (15% fat)

- 1/3 cup quick-cooking oats
- 1 medium onion, chopped very fine (see note)
- 1 Tbsp. vegetable oil, for frying onion
- 2 Tbsp. stick margarine, for frying meatballs

Gravy:

- 1 14-oz. can Health Valley Fat Free Beef Broth
- 1/2 tsp. ground nutmeg
- 1/4 tsp. ground allspice
- 1/2 tsp. dried dill weed
- 1/2 tsp. salt
- 1 Tbsp. white wine (optional)
- 1/2 cup water, divided
- 3 Tbsp. cornstarch
- 1/3 cup heavy cream

Instructions

1. In a small dish whisk together the egg, nutmeg, allspice and salt for the meatballs. Add to the ground beef and quick oats. Mix well and set aside. In a large skillet, fry the onion in a little oil until all the bits are translucent and few are starting to brown. Remove the skillet from the heat. Mix the onion into the meat and form meatballs, about an inch to an inch-and-a-half across. Place on a plate and set aside for the moment.

2. In a covered soup pot heat the beef broth, nutmeg, allspice, dill, salt(and wine if desired) to a simmer. Reheat the skillet and brown the meatballs in margarine. As they are browned, add to the simmering soup. Remove the skillet from heat, add 1/4 cup of the

water and stir to scrape up the browned bits. Pour into the simmering liquid. Let the liquid and meatballs simmer covered for 8 minutes.

3. In a small dish add the remaining 1/4 cup water to the cornstarch and blend until smooth. Stir in the cream. Add the cream mixture all at once to the simmering meatballs while carefully stirring. Over low heat allow the gravy to thicken and reheat (but don't allow it to boil). Serve over hot cooked noodles.

Fresh Yellow Tomato Soup

Servings: 3

Ingredients

- 1 Tbsp. extra virgin olive oil
- 1 medium onion, peeled and diced OR
- 2 Tbsp. dried minced onions (see note below)
- 2 teaspoons flour
- 1 cup water (reserved from cooking tomatoes)
- 2 lbs. ripe yellow low-acid tomatoes
- 2 cloves garlic, peeled and minced
- 1 teaspoon Italian seasoning (see note below)
- 1 teaspoon sugar
- 1/2 teaspoon salt
- 1/2 teaspoon pepper, optional

Instructions

1. In a large pot cover tomatoes with water and boil for 10 to 15 minutes. Drain and save 1 cup of the water.

Remove stem and core of tomatoes, then cut into large chunks. Puree tomatoes (skins and all) in batches.

2. Strain the tomato puree into a bowl, pressing as much pulp as you can through a strainer, leaving the seeds.

3. Heat oil in a large saucepan. When it is hot, add the onion and saute it over medium heat for 3 to 4 minutes until translucent. (If you are using dried onions, add them later). Add flour to the onions, mix well and cook another minute. Add garlic and saute for one minute. Add the tomato puree, 1 cup of the reserved water, and remaining ingredients. Mix well.

4. Bring soup to a boil then reduce heat. Cover an simmer for 20 minutes. Adjust seasoning to taste. Serve

immediately or cool, cover and refrigerate. Reheat when ready to serve.

Honey Garlic Chicken

Ingredients

- 4 Bone-in Chicken Thighs
- Kosher Salt, to taste
- Ground Black Pepper, to taste (if tolerated)
- 1 Tablespoon Unsalted Butter
- 2 Tablespoons Chopped Garlic
- 1 teaspoon Dried Thyme
- 1/3 Cup Honey
- 1 Pound Green Beans, trimmed
- 1 Pound other vegetable
- 1 Lemon (Optional), zested and juiced (start with half of the zest and juice

and add more to taste, if needed), if tolerated

Instructions

1. Preheat your oven to 400°F/200°C. Season the chicken thighs with salt and pepper on both sides. Heat a large ovenproof skillet over medium heat and add 1 tablespoon of butter. Add the seasoned chicken, skin-side down, and sear on both sides until it's golden brown, about 3-5 minutes per side. Remove the chicken thighs and set them aside.

2. Drain off the excess fat, leaving about 1 tablespoon in the pan, and return the skillet to medium heat. Add the garlic and cook, stirring constantly, until fragrant, about 1 minute. Add the

dried thyme, honey, and lemon zest and juice (if using). Bring the sauce to a simmer and stir to combine. Reduce the heat to low.

3. Return the chicken to the pan and coat each piece with the sauce. Move the chicken to one side of the pan and add the green beans and other vegetable to the open space in the pan. Transfer the skillet to the oven and bake it until the chicken is cooked through, about 20-25 minutes.

4. Allow the chicken to rest for a few minutes before serving.

Slow Cooker Roast Beef

Ingredients

- 3 to 4 pound beef roast, visible fat trimmed
- 4 medium potatoes, peeled and halved (can substitute sweet potatoes)
- 3 carrots, peeled and cut into 2-inch pieces
- 2 stalks of celery, cut into 1/2-inch pieces
- 1 medium onion, quartered, if tolerated
- 1/2 c. boiling water
- 1 T. minced garlic
- 1 t. salt
- 1/2 t. pepper, if tolerated
- 2 t. dried basil

Instructions

1. Layer roast and vegetables in a 3 qt slow cooker.

2. Add water. Sprinkle in garlic, salt, pepper, and basil.

3. Cook on medium for 6 to 8 hours or on high for 4 to 6 hours. Temperature of roast at its center should be a minimum of 145°.

Soft Chicken Tacos with Roasted Red Pepper and Corn

Servings: 6

Ingredients

- 1 T. olive oil
- ½ c. chopped onion
- 1 garlic clove, peeled and chopped (optional, as tolerated)
- ½ c. chopped roasted sweet red pepper

- 1 ½ c. cooked, shredded chicken (may substitute ground meat)
- ½ t. cumin
- ½ t. paprika
- 1 t. chopped oregano
- Salt and pepper to taste
- ½ c. roasted sweet red pepper, chopped and chilled
- ½ c. corn (for more flavor, use kernels from grilled corn on the cob. Chill before using.)
- ½ c. canned black beans, drained and rinsed
- ½ c. cubed cucumber
- ¼ c. chopped onion (if tolerated)
- 2 t. pear juice
- 1 t. olive oil
- 1 t. chopped cilantro
- ¼ t. lime zest

- 1 t. chopped oregano
- 6 small corn or flour soft tortillas
- Lettuce
- Cheese
- 1 avocado cut into slices

Instructions

1. Heat olive oil in skillet over medium heat. Add first ½ c. onions, garlic, and first ½ c. red peppers, cooking until slightly browned and caramelized. Add shredded chicken, cumin, paprika, oregano, salt, and pepper and heat until cooked through.

2. While meat mixture is heating, combine second ½ c. red pepper, corn, black beans, cucumbers, second ½ c. onions, pear juice, oil, cilantro, lime zest, and oregano to make salsa.

44

3. To warm and soften tortillas, place two between paper towels and heat for 20 seconds in the microwave. Fill with meat mixture. Top with lettuce, cheese, salsa, and avocado slices. Enjoy!

Beans With Rosemary And Pine Nuts

Servings: 4

Ingredients

- 2 cups frozen green beans
- 1 Tbsp. margarine
- 1 Tbsp. olive oil
- 1/2 tsp. dried rosemary, slightly crushed
- 1/8 tsp. garlic powder
- 1 dash salt

- 2 Tbsp. pine nuts

Instructions

1. Cook green beans, drain and set aside. In skillet, melt margarine over low to medium heat and add olive oil.
2. Stir in garlic powder, salt, and rosemary.
3. Add green beans and pine nuts. Cook, stirring over medium heat until beans and pine nuts are heated through and thoroughly coated with oil and margarine mixture.
4. Turn into a serving bowl.

Orange-Almond Yams

Servings: 8

Ingredients

- 3 lbs. sweet potatoes, cooked; or two 15-oz cans cooked yams
- 1 cup brown sugar, packed
- 2 Tbsp. cornstarch
- 1/4 tsp. salt
- 1/4 tsp. ground cinnamon
- 1 cup apricot nectar
- 1/2 cup hot water
- 3 tsp. grated orange peel
- 1 Tbsp. margarine
- 1/2 cup sliced almonds

Instructions

1. Place cooked, sliced yams or sweet potatoes in a 13 x 9 x 2-inch pan. Preheat oven to 350 degrees F.
2. In a saucepan combine brown sugar, cornstarch, salt and cinnamon. Stir in

apricot nectar, hot water and orange peel.

3. Bring to a boil and, stirring constantly, cook for two minutes.

4. Remove from heat; stir in margarine and almonds. Pour over yams. Bake, uncovered, at 350 degrees for 20-25 minutes.

Asparagus Soup

Ingredients

- 1 ½ pounds fresh asparagus, rinsed
- 4 cups MSG free chicken broth (Swanson's)
- Bowl of ice water
- 2 T. unsalted butter or olive oil

- ½ cup minced leek whites (usually well tolerated by people with interstitial cystitis)
- 1 tsp. minced garlic
- ¼ tsp. salt
- Dash or two white pepper (if tolerated)
- ½ cup heavy cream or evaporated milk
- Grated Parmesan cheese (optional garnish)

Instructions

1. Cut tips from the asparagus, about 1 to 1 ½ inches in length and set aside. Cut off woody ends of stalks at about 1 ½ inches, also setting aside separately. Cut the remaining stalks into ½ inch pieces. Bring stock to a boil in medium

stock pot. Add the woody end stems, simmering for 20 minutes to infuse with asparagus flavor. Use slotted spoon to remove and discard woody stems.

2. Blanch asparagus tips for 1 minute in steaming broth, using a slotted spoon, remove to bowl of ice water to stop cooking. Remove from ice water to paper towel. Set aside broth.

3. In another medium stockpot, melt the butter or heat olive oil over medium-high heat. Add leek whites, cooking about 3 minutes until tender. Add garlic, cooking for additional minute. Add the tender chopped asparagus stalks, salt, and pepper. Continue to stir and cook for additional 2 minutes. Add the broth from first pot and

simmer until the asparagus is tender, about 20 minutes. Remove from the heat.

4. Puree soup using blender, immersion blender, or food processor. Return to stock pot and add cream and half of the blanched asparagus tips, warming soup for about 2 more minutes. Serve in large soup bowl. Garnish with a few of the remaining asparagus tips and Parmesan cheese. Enjoy!

No Cheese Pesto Sauce for Pasta

Ingredients

- 3 c. fresh basil leaves
- 1 c. fresh parsley sprig
- 4 garlic cloves, crushed
- 4 T. olive oil

- 3 T. toasted pine nuts
- Pepper, if tolerated, to taste

Instructions

1. Use food processor to chop basil and parsley.
2. Add garlic and olive oil; process another 20 seconds.
3. Add pine nuts and finish processing. Use as topping for pasta or baked potatoes, or as a garnish for chicken.

Slow Cooker Chicken Noodle Soup

Ingredients

- 3 boneless, skinless chicken breasts
- 4 medium carrots, peeled and sliced into coins

- 3 stalks celery, cut into small, bite-sized pieces
- 1 medium sweet onion, diced
- 3 to 4 cloves garlic, minced
- 2 tablespoons butter or olive oil
- 1 teaspoon poultry seasoning (MSG-free)
- 6 cups MSG free chicken broth (Swanson's is available almost everywhere)
- ½ teaspoon of salt
- ¼ teaspoon of black pepper (if tolerated)
- 1 ½ cupped cooked eggs noodles

Instructions

1. Add whole chicken breasts to pre-heated, 5 to 6 quart slow cooker. Add

carrots, celery, onion, garlic, broth, and seasonings.

2. Cover and cook on low heat for 6 to 8 hours or until chicken breasts reach an internal temperature of 165 degrees F. Remove chicken breasts.

3. Chop into bite sized pieces and return to soup mixture. Add cooked noodles. Cook for an additional 30 minutes. Serve hot.Slow C

Chicken and White Bean Soup

Servings: 6

Ingredients

- 2 teaspoon extra-virgin olive oil
- 2 leeks, white and light green parts only, cut into 1/4-inch rounds

- 1/2 teaspoon dried sage
- 3 14-ounce cans reduced salt chicken broth
- 1 15-ounce can cannellini beans, rinsed
- 3 boneless chicken breasts, baked and shredded

Instructions

1. Heat oil in large pot over medium high heat.
2. Add leeks and cook, stirring until soft (about 3 minutes).
3. Stir in sage and keep cooking until aromatic (about 30 seconds).
4. Stir in broth, raise heat to high, cover and bring to a boil.
5. Add beans and chicken and cook until heated through (about 3 minutes).
6. Serve hot.

Slow Cooker Beef Stew

Ingredients

- 2 lbs. beef chuck

- 1 tsp. paprika

- 1 1/2 tsp. salt

- 1/2 tsp. pepper

- 1/3 cup all purpose flour

- 3 Tbsp. olive oil or shortening

- 1 medium white onion (if tolerated), sliced thinly

- 1 clove garlic, chopped

- 1/2 pound small mushrooms whole or cut in halves

- 1 pound small white potatoes, cut into quarters

- 1/2 package baby cut organic carrots

- 2-3 cups organic beef broth, low salt (no msg please)
- fresh thyme springs

Instructions

1. Cut beef into bite size pieces. Toss with paprika, salt and pepper and flour, the shake off excess flour. Heat oil to medium high in your slow cooker and brown meat. Cook until browned on all sides.

2. Add in sliced onions, chopped garlic, carrots, mushrooms and potatoes and continue to saute for five minutes.

3. Add two to three cups of beef broth and fresh thyme. Simmer on low for 6-8 hours or until meat and veggies are tender. If you would prefer a gravy like sauce, remove 1/2 cup of sauce

from the slow cooker. Stir (or whisk) in 1/4 cup flour into the 1/2 cup sauce until no clumps remain. Stir back into the slow cooker and cook for an additional five or ten minutes until the sauce thickens.

Savory Chicken and Broccoli Casserole

Ingredients

- 6 ounces egg noodles (without problem ingredients)
- 3 tablespoons butter
- 1 yellow onion, chopped (if tolerated)
- 1/4 cup all-purpose flour
- 1 1/2 cups chicken broth (without problem ingredients)
- 3/4 cup milk
- salt and pepper to taste (if tolerated)

- 5 cups cooked, shredded chicken breast meat
- 1 (10 ounce) package chopped frozen broccoli, thawed
- 1 cup shredded Cheddar cheese
- 1 cup shredded provolone cheese (if tolerated)

Instructions

1. Ring a large pot of lightly salted water to a boil. Add pasta and cook for 6 to 8 minutes or until al dente; drain. Preheat oven to 400 degrees F (200 degrees C.) Grease a 9x13 inch casserole dish.

2. Melt butter in a large saucepan over medium heat. Sauté onion until tender, about 3 minutes. Mix in flour. Gradually stir in chicken broth. Slowly

stir in milk, and cook, stirring, until sauce begins to thicken. Season with salt and pepper.

3. Place cooked noodles in the bottom of casserole dish. Arrange cooked chicken in an even layer over noodles. Place broccoli over the chicken. Pour sauce evenly over the broccoli. Combine cheeses, and sprinkle half over the casserole.

4. Bake in preheated oven for 20 minutes, or until the cheese melts. Remove from oven, and sprinkle with remaining cheese. Allow to set for 5 minutes, until cheese melts.

Mini Chicken Pot Pies

Ingredients

- 1 tablespoon vegetable oil
- 1 lb boneless skinless chicken breasts, cut into bite-size pieces (or use leftover cooked chicken)
- 1 medium onion (1/2 cup), chopped (if tolerated)
- 1/2 cup chicken broth (without problem ingredients)
- 1 cup frozen peas and carrots
- 1/2 teaspoon salt
- 1/4 teaspoon pepper (if tolerated)
- 1/4 teaspoon ground thyme
- 1 cup shredded Cheddar cheese (4 oz)

Baking Mixture

- 1/2 cup Original Bisquick™ mix
- 1/2 cup milk
- 2 eggs

Instructions

1. Heat oven to 375°F. Spray 12 regular-size muffin cups with cooking spray.

2. In 10-inch nonstick skillet, heat oil over medium-high heat. Cook chicken in oil 5 to 7 minutes, stirring occasionally, until chicken is no longer pink in center. Add onion and chicken broth; heat to simmering. Add frozen vegetables and seasonings. Heat until hot, stirring occasionally until almost all liquid is absorbed. Cool 5 minutes; stir in cheese.

3. In medium bowl, stir baking mixture ingredients with whisk or fork until blended. Spoon 1 scant tablespoon baking mixture into each muffin cup. Top with about 1/4 cup chicken mixture. Spoon 1 tablespoon baking

mixture onto chicken mixture in each muffin cup.

4. Bake 25 to 30 minutes or until toothpick inserted in center comes out clean. Cool 5 minutes. With thin knife, loosen sides of pies from pan; remove from pan and place top sides up on cooling rack. Cool 10 minutes longer, and serve.

Creamy Garlic Herb Mushroom Spaghetti

Servings: 4

Ingredients

- 8 ounces whole wheat pasta (spaghetti, linguine, etc.)
- 4 tablespoons butter, divided

- 3 cloves garlic, minced, divided
- 16 ounces fresh mushrooms, sliced
- 2 tablespoons flour (or whole wheat flour)
- 1 teaspoon herbes de provence
- 1 1/2 cups milk
- salt and pepper to taste
- 3 tablespoons olive oil
- additional 1/4 cup water, broth, milk or cream (optional)
- 1/4 cup fresh parsley (more to taste)

Instructions

1. **Pasta:** Cook the pasta according to package directions. Set aside and toss with a little oil to prevent sticking.
2. **Mushrooms:** Melt 2 tablespoons of butter over medium high heat. Add one clove of the garlic and saute for a

minute until fragrant. Add the mushrooms and sauté for 5-10 minutes, until golden brown and softened. Set aside.

3. **Sauce:** Add the remaining 2 tablespoons of butter to the pan and melt again over medium high heat. Add the garlic and saute for a minute until fragrant. Add the flour and herbes de provence. Stir fry for a minute to cook out the flour taste. Add the milk slowly, whisking to incorporate. Let the mixture simmer until thickened. Season with salt and pepper.

4. **Assemble:** Toss the sauce, pasta, and mushrooms together. Add the olive oil and water as needed to keep the sauce

from getting too thick. Stir in the parsley just before serving

Oven-Fried Panko Crusted Chicken Drumsticks

Ingredients

- 6 chicken drumsticks
- 1 egg
- 1 tablespoons water
- 4 tablespoons butter
- 1 cup panko breadcrumbs
- 2 tablespoons grated parmesan cheese
- 1/2 tsp kosher salt
- 1/2 tsp smoked paprika
- 1/4 tsp garlic powder
- 1/4 tsp onion powder
- 1/4 tsp dried oregano
- 1/4 tsp dried basil

- 1/4 tsp fresh ground black pepper

Instructions

1. Preheat your oven to 425 degrees F. Put the butter in your cast iron skillet and place it in the oven to melt.

2. Meanwhile, in a shallow dish whisk together the egg and the water. In another shallow dish, combine the breadcrumbs, parmesan, salt, paprika, garlic powder, onion powder, oregano, basil and black pepper.

3. Dip the drumsticks in the egg mixture followed by the breadcrumb mixture, pressing the coating firmly onto each piece. Put the drumsticks into the pan of melted butter and drizzle them with olive oil.

4. Bake the chicken for 30 minutes, flip then continue to bake for an additional 15 minutes.

Roasted Potatoes

Ingredients

- 2 Lbs of white or yellow potatoes (peeled or unpeeled), cut into 1/2 inch pieces. (Sometimes russet potatoes work o.k. but tend not to hold their shape as well)
- 2 Tbsp melted butter
- 2 Tbsp olive oil
- 2 tsp dried parsley
- 1 tsp paprika (smoked paprika is really good here)
- 1/2 tsp salt

- 1/4 to 1/2 tsp of freshly ground black pepper (to taste)
- 1/4 tsp of garlic powder (or cut up several garlic cloves and mix in)

Instructions

1. Preheat oven to 425°F. Place potatoes in a 9 x 13 pan.
2. Pour melted butter and olive oil over potatoes and add the remaining ingredients. Stir together until potatoes are evenly coated.
3. Place in oven and and bake, stirring every 15 minutes (so they evenly crisp and don't stick to pan), until potatoes are tender and starting to brown in spots and get crispy. This will take about 45-55 min.

Lump Free Homemade Gravy

Ingredients

- 2 cups roast beef drippings.
- handful of ice cubes
- 2 Tablespoons Cornstarch
- 1/4 cup cold water
- Salt and pepper to taste
- Onion powder and Garlic pepper to taste (optional)

Instructions

1. Toss ice cubes into beef drippings
2. Combine Cornstarch and cold water in sauce pan and whisk until smooth
3. lightly skim solidified fat from the top of the beef drippings
4. Combine beef drippings with cornstarch mixture in sauce pan.
5. Add seasonings

6. Turn to medium high and heat until a boil, stirring constantly

7. Cook at a boil for 1 minute or until consistency of your choice

8. Remove from heat and serve.

Butternut Squash and Kale Lasagna

Servings: 6-8

Ingredients

- 2 Tbsp olive oil
- 1 medium butternut squash, peeled and cut into small cubes
- 1 Tbsp brown sugar
- Sea salt and fresh ground black pepper
- 3 cloves fresh garlic, peeled and diced
- 1/4 tsp nutmeg (if tolerated although in this quantity, may not be a problem)

- 2 tsps fresh thyme, chopped
- 1 bunch kale, washed, stems removed and chopped or a large container of baby spinach washed, stems removed and chopped
- (about 4 cups)
- 1 pound low-fat ricotta cheese
- another 1/2 tsp nutmeg
- 6 fresh sage sprigs, chopped and 2 more for topping
- Mozzarella cheese, low-fat or regular, shredded to make 1/2 cup plus some to sprinkle on top if desired
- 1 cup fresh pecorino cheese, grated (or fresh grated parmesan) plus 2-3 Tbsp to sprinkle on top
- 1/3 cup low-fat milk
- 1 pound no-boil lasagna noodles, whole wheat (or 1 pound pasta)

- 2 Tbsp pumpkin seeds to sprinkle on top

Instructions

1. Preheat oven to 400 degrees. Heat olive oil in a large skillet over medium heat. Add butternut squash and sprinkle with brown sugar and season with sea salt and fresh ground pepper. Cook for 10-15 minutes stirring frequently to avoid burning until browned. Add garlic, nutmeg, and thyme, cook 5 minutes more.
2. Remove from heat and add kale, cover and let sit 10 minutes until kale wilts.
3. In a large bowl mix ricotta cheese with remaining 1/2 tsp nutmeg, sage, mozzarella cheese, pecorino or

parmesan cheese and milk. Season with salt and pepper.

4. Heavily spray or butter a 9 by 13 baking dish and layer with 1/3 of the lasagna noodles. Add 1/3 of the kale/squash mixture layered over the noodles. Add 1/3 of the cheese mixture and drizzle with a little olive oil. Repeat the layering 2 more times or until all is used. Drizzle a little olive oil over top. Sprinkle with pecorino or parmesan and sage leaves as the top layer. If you like a browned, crunchy top, add a final topping of mozzarella after initial baking and bake 10 more minutes or until mozzarella is browned.

5. Cover with foil sprayed with cooking spray and refrigerate up to 3 days. Or

bake immediately at 400 degrees for 35-45 minutes and uncovered 10 more if topping with mozzarella. If you are baking after refrigeration, add 15-20 minutes to baking time.

6. Sprinkle with pumpkin seeds (or pine nuts) and serve.

Turkey Pot pies

Servings: 4

Ingredients

- 4 T butter
- 1 T diced garlic
- 2 medium carrots, peeled and thinly sliced
- 1 stick of celery, thinly sliced
- salt and pepper

- 4 T flour
- 2 1/2 cups turkey, chicken or vegetable broth (low sodium, organic)
- 1/4 cup heavy cream or milk
- 3/4 tsp dried or 2 tsp fresh thyme, chopped
- 1 1/2 cups cooked, shredded skinless turkey or chicken meat (organic, broth-free or preservative free)
- 1/2 cup peas
- 2 T chopped fresh parsley
- 1 sheet frozen puff pastry, thawed (some contain citric acid low on the ingredient list – a try-it item)
- 1 large egg

Instructions

1. Warm butter in a large saucepan on low heat. Add garlic, carrot and celery,

sprinkle with salt and pepper and cook, stirring occasionally until tender 10 min.

2. Sprinkle with flour and cook 3 min, stirring constantly. Pour in broth and cream/milk. Stir in thyme. Bring to a simmer over medium heat. Reduce heat and gently simmer 10 min until thick and stir to prevent sticking.

3. Remove from heat. Stir in chicken or turkey, peas and parsley. Divide into 4 8 ounce ramekins. Place on rimmed, foil-covered baking sheet.

4. Place puff pastry on lightly floured surface. Slice into 4 inch squares and place over ramekins.

5. Whisk egg and 1 T water in a small bowl. Brush pastry tops with egg mixture.

6. Bake until golden and bubbly about 35 minutes in 375 degree oven. Let stand 5 min then serve.

Slow Cooker Sweet Potato Soup

Servings: 4

Ingredients

- 3 lbs. sweet potatoes, roughly chopped and peeled or not
- 1 sweet onion, chopped (if tolerated or omit)
- 2 stalks of sliced celery
- 2 chopped medium carrots
- 1-2 Tbsp minced fresh garlic
- 5 cups of organic low sodium chicken or vegetable stock
- 1 cup of coconut milk

- Sea salt and freshly ground pepper or cinnamon, all-spice or nutmeg (if tolerated) to taste

Instructions

1. Place all ingredients except the coconut milk in a slow cooker.
2. Season to taste with salt and pepper. Cover and cook on low 6 hours or on high for 4 hours.
3. Puree everything in a blender or leave chunky.
4. Add coconut milk, stir thoroughly and cook another 30 minutes.
5. Adjust seasoning and serve warm with a sprig of parsley for color.

White Bean Chicken Chili

Servings: 6

Ingredients

- 1 tablespoon olive oil
- 1 cup chopped sweet onion (if tolerated)
- 1 cup chopped celery
- 2 sweet bell peppers cored and chopped (red, yellow or orange or green if tolerated)
- 1 pound ground lean chicken or turkey with no preservatives (for vegetarian chili substitute 1 can of beans and 1 cup of corn)
- It is also possible to use 2 cups grilled chicken breast or turkey tenderloin instead of ground
- 1 tablespoon minced garlic

- 1 tablespoon all-purpose flour
- 1 teaspoon ground cumin (if tolerated or substitute dried basil)
- 1 teaspoon dried oregano
- 2 cups chicken or vegetable broth low-sodium or with no preservatives
- 2 15 ounce cans white beans drained and rinsed (mash one can of beans for thicker chili)
- 1/2 cup low-fat sour cream or plain yogurt (if tolerated)
- salt and pepper to taste
- shredded mild cheddar cheese for topping and/or can chopped mild green chilis if tolerated

Instructions

1. In a large pot over medium heat warm the oil. Add chopped veggies and

sautee for 5 min. Add chicken or turkey and cook through at least 5 minutes. Omit for vegetarian chili.

2. Add the garlic, flour, cumin (or basil) and oregano. Cook, stirring over low heat 2 minutes. Add the broth while stirring. Increase heat and bring to a boil stirring occasionally. Reduce heat to simmering and cook 10 minutes longer.

3. Add the beans and simmer another 10 minutes. Mash 1 can of the beans for thicker chili. Add a third can of beans and corn for vegetarian chili.

4. Stir in sour cream or yogurt. Season with salt and pepper.

5. Ladle into bowls and top with shredded cheddar and green chilis. May be served over rice, quinoa or

other cooked grains. Add a warm piece of corn bread for a more hearty meal.

Butternut Squash Mac 'n Cheese

Ingredients

- 1/2 butternut squash, peeled and chopped (yields: 3.5 cups raw)
- 3/4 cup raw cashews
- 1 cup milk, or more to thin out
- 3 garlic cloves
- 1 tsp lemon zest
- 2 tsp kosher salt, or to taste
- 6-7 tbsp Nutritional yeast (provides the cheesy consistency)
- 1/2 tsp or a bit more of dried Italian seasoning

- 1/4-1/2 tsp Tumeric powder, if tolerated optional (gives the orangey colour)
- Freshly ground black pepper, to taste if tolerated
- Your pasta of choice (I used ~450 grams/4.5 cups dry penne for the casserole) + mix-ins

Instructions

1. Preheat oven to 350 degrees F and line a baking sheet. In a bowl, season chopped squash with some oil (~1 tsp) and kosher salt (couple pinches) and stir. Add to baking sheet and roast in oven for 40 minutes, flipping once half way through baking.
2. If making the baked casserole: Process 1 slice of bread + 1 tbsp nutritiional

yeast until crumbs form in a food processor. Set aside. If you plan on enjoying it straight from the pot you can skip this step.

3. Assemble your cheese sauce ingredients (cashews, milk, garlic, lemon zest, salt, nutritional yeast, pepper, mustard, seasonings) and add just the cashews to food processor. Process until a fine crumb forms similar to corn meal. Now add in the rest of the cheese sauce ingredients and process until smooth. Leave the sauce in the processor as you will be adding the squash.

4. Cook your pasta according to package directions. When squash is finished roasting, add it to the food processor or blender and blend it with the cheese

sauce until smooth. Adjust to taste. The sauce will thicken up with time. If at any point the sauce becomes too thick, you can add a bit of milk to thin it out.

5. Drain and rinse pasta with cold water. Now add the pasta back into the same pot and add your desired amount of cheese sauce on top. Stir well. Add in any desired mix-ins like peas or broccoli. You can either heat this up in the pot, or pour it into a casserole dish (I used a 4 cup dish), sprinkle on breadcrumbs + paprika, and bake it at 350 for about 20-25 minutes. The casserole will serve about 4 people if you use 450 grams dry macaroni or penne. Store any leftover sauce in the fridge and use within a few days.

Red Lentil and Squash Stew

Servings: 4

Ingredients

- 1 tsp Extra virgin olive oil
- 1 sweet onion, chopped (if tolerated)
- 3 garlic cloves, minced
- 1 tbsp turmeric (if tolerated), or more to taste
- 1 carton broth (4 cups)
- 1 cup red lentils
- 3 cups cooked butternut squash
- 1 cup greens of choice
- Fresh grated ginger, to taste (optional)
- Kosher salt & black pepper, to taste (I used about 1/2 tsp salt)

Instructions

1. In a large pot, add olive oil and chopped onion and minced garlic. Saute for about 5 minutes over low-medium heat.

2. Stir in turmeric and cook another couple minutes. Add broth and lentils and bring to a boil. Reduce heat and cook for 10 minutes.

3. Stir in cooked butternut squash and greens of choice. Cook over medium heat for about 5-8 minutes. Season with salt, pepper, and add some freshly grated ginger to taste.

Made in United States
North Haven, CT
29 June 2022